Copyright 2015
Mark Thorsell

Dedication

This is dedicated to my wife, Marcia.

Sweetie,
Parkinson's Disease may have entered my

brain, but we both
got it.
 We both have to deal
with it every day.
I think you have the
more difficult task.
Thank you for
walking, (shuffling),
this journey with me.
A journey neither of
us chose.
Even though I may
lose much of my
ability to show it, I

will love you literally
forever.

FORWARD

I am a man living in the United States in the 21st century. I am in my early 60's. I'm a husband, father, grandfather, son, brother, father in law, uncle, friend, follower of Jesus and I have Parkinson's Disease. Because I have Parkinson's, my world has changed color. Much of the world doesn't look good this color. Some things just look different. Things are being taken away. The ability to speak clearly is one example. My sense of smell is another. The ability to walk normally is another. Things are being added. Having a jaw that has a mind of its own and moves when it wants to. I now walk with a cane. These things were not offered to me and are not welcomed. Since my diagnosis, I discovered I like to write. I like the process of thinking about an idea and writing it down. I don't believe it is something I desired to do or did before my diagnosis. But now it's almost a compulsion. They say that compulsive behavior is part of P.D. It could be from the disease or the medications. Wherever it comes from, I enjoy writing.

I must apologize in advance. What you are about to read is flawed. The fact that I started writing so late in life means I haven't had a lot of practice or education in the correct way to structure sentences. Despite spell check, spelling will not be perfect. I will try hard not to mix my

metaphors or dangle my participles. But as hard as I will try, it will happen.
So, I'm sorry.

With that out of the way, I think I'll write something.

What Defines Us

Having to live with something like Parkinson's Disease becomes something that defines you. We are all defined by different things...things we have no control over, like being tall or short, shy or extroverted, attractive or less attractive, coordinated or uncoordinated. Other things that define us we create ourselves... being mean or kind, patient or impatient, neat or dirty, generous or stingy.

Up until 2009, I was defined by being tall, being a son and a brother, being a husband and father, my wife would say "opinionated", and many other things. Then, along came Parkinson's.

For the first few years, it was just a footnote in my story.

Few people noticed any outward signs and I hardly felt its presence. But now it's becoming a Chapter Title. Most people see the outward signs that something is wrong. I feel it with every movement I make. I am increasingly being defined as a man with Parkinson's Disease.

Everyone is defined by many things. The primary definitions come from outward appearance, where we came from and where we have been, choices we have made along the way and what has happened to us on our journey through life. Very few live their entire life defined by the same things all the way through. Usually something comes along, invited or uninvited, that changes our lives and the way others see us.

I worked for the same company for 31 years. That company

was started by a man that went from growing up poor to becoming very successful, both in business and personally. Along his journey, he was with the 82nd Airborne, a fireman, built a very successful plumbing company employing over 100 plumbers at its peak, (also obtaining the first plumbing license ever issued by Orange County, Fl, license #001). Built an oil and gas drilling company with wells in Ohio, Oklahoma and Texas, and then started a commercial real estate company with his three sons that ultimately changed the face of Orlando.

He was defined by things like husband, father, grandfather, great grandfather, honest, successful, hard working, generous and a Christian Man.

Before the words Parkinson's Disease ever crossed my mind, this strong man began to talk about feeling weakness and a shaking on one side of his body. As time went by, the symptoms increased and spread to other parts of his body, to the point where he had to make the hard decision to stop driving. The only bright spot in that decision was for me. I was given the privilege of driving him for the next year. To be able to spend that much time alone with that great man was wonderful. The stories and wisdom he shared are priceless.

It broke my heart to witness the slow decline he had to endure. He was a great example of someone coping with and rising above adversity. It was hard for me when he reached the point of not going into the office anymore. Fortunately, I was able to still see him every week up to and including the day he went Home.

I don't think they ever
called what he had
Parkinson's Disease,
but 7 years ago, when
those words were
first used to define
me, I have seen many
of the same
symptoms in me that
I saw in him. But
because of what I
learned from being
with him and his
example, I am better

prepared for my
journey Home.

As I live this chapter
of my life, I will more
and more be
described as a man
with Parkinson's
Disease. Despite that,
I'm going to work
hard at making that
definition of me
follow behind
definitions like good

husband, good father and grandfather, good friend, a man that loves God and lives well despite adversity.

My Adversary

I thought I would say
a few more words
about this "thing"
that lives with me.
Years ago he snuck up
on me. So, quiet and
sneaky that for a long
time, I didn't even
know he was there.

He did leave little hints from time to time, but I didn't realize it was him. Like when he stole my sense of smell. I blamed it on a stinky job I was asked to do. It was so smelly, I thought my brain just said, "That's it, no more smelling for you". Along with my sense of smell, he stole my sense of taste. Didn't steal it altogether, but altered the taste of everything.

Then he stole my left arms ability to swing when I walk. It just kind of hangs there, ignoring what the rest of my body is doing.

He started to take my voice. My kids would ask me to scream, and out would come this low weird sound. We all laughed and they would ask me to do it again. It was funny until those around me started having trouble hearing what I would say.

He would also give me gifts. He gave me the gift of a constantly runny nose. (There are certain things you have with you all the time, your underwear, your cell phone, etc. To my things to always carry, I've added a handful of paper towels. The problem is I leave a rolled-up paper towel everywhere I go. Drives my family and co-workers nuts. I tell them the towels are not left, they are staged.)

Then the constant sleepiness and fatigue began.

The final straw was when he stole my joy. The other things he stole from me I could take, but not my joy. That was too much.

What I didn't know was this "thing" was waging a war against my brain, and my brain was losing.

I went to see a doctor that people I trust said would know what was happening to me. This doctor gave the "thing", the intruder and thief a name, Parkinson's Disease. It was like giving a face to an enemy. The doctor not only gave my adversary an identity, he provided me with weapons to fight him with. Unfortunately, at this stage of the battle, the weapons are mostly defensive. But people are working day and night on offensive weapons.

Fortunately, armed with the defensive weapons and my willingness to fight, I can keep this creep at bay, at least for a while.

But it is a fight. My enemy never sleeps. He doesn't just steal things suddenly. He takes them and slowly carries them beyond my reach.

Like riding a motorcycle or bicycle. Using my hands. Saying what I want loudly and clearly. Running. Playing video games. Standing for more than a short time. Holding my grandson. But there are some things the enemy can never touch. The love of and for my wife.

The love of and for my kids and all my family. The love of and for my friends. The love of and for God.
These are things that will be here after he's gone.

That gives me Joy!

The Cost of Forgiveness

I believe forgiveness is one of the most powerful actions in the universe.

The story is told that God decided to create a man. God

told the man not to do something. The man did it anyway. Because of this wrong, all the men that came from that man did wrong.

God had a choice. Allow all men to die being wrong, or forgive them. Either choice came at a cost.

God created man for relationship with Him. If He chose to let men die without His forgiveness, there would be no relationship. If He chose to forgive, it would cost Him His Son.

Many times, in life we have a choice. The choice to forgive or

remain wronged.
Both choices still have
a cost.

A husband and wife
have two young
children. They are a
happy family. One
day the wife
overhears a phone
conversation
between her husband
and a co-worker.
Things are said that

lead her to believe her husband is having an affair. She tries to dismiss it, but over time it becomes clear that the affair is real. She confronts him. He confesses. He promises her that he will end it. He asks for her forgiveness.

She now has a choice. Both choices have a

cost. She has been wronged. She can choose to not forgive him. The costs are a broken home, children that are damaged forever, the costs that come with not following God's directive to forgive, a quenched Spirit, a hardened heart, the list goes on and on.

If she chooses to forgive him, there are also costs.... humiliation that comes with betrayal, having to build trust, having to battle suspicion, mourning the loss of what they had built together.

But the rewards of forgiveness are... The chance to rebuild a life together, undamaged and happy children, the joy and peace of following God, the Spirit being allowed to work in her family, and the heritage enabled by forgiveness that will go on for generations.

Withholding forgiveness has no rewards.

They Look Like Trees

The story is told of a man that was born blind. Jesus put his hands on the man's eyes and then asked the man, "Can you see?" The man replied, "Yes, but the men I see look like trees walking around." Jesus then placed his hands on the man's eyes a second time. This time the man could see everything clearly.

I have always been puzzled by this story. Why didn't the man see clearly after the first time Jesus placed

His hands on him?
Wasn't there enough
healing power in His
first touch? There is
no doubt in my mind
that Jesus was able to
heal the man totally
even without
touching him. I
believe the man
needed two healings.
Why two healings?

I remember a news article about people that had never been able to see suddenly getting the ability to see by a medical procedure. Everything they knew about the world they had learned without sight. They had discovered the world by touch, taste, smell and hearing. What I found interesting was that with a large number of these people, once they gained their sight, what they saw did not make any sense to them. They couldn't recognize anything. The world they had grown to know through their other senses was nothing like the world they now could see. The world became so confusing and distressing that many of them covered their eyes and some even asked that their ability to see be removed. The conclusion of the doctors was that you must heal the mind along with giving the ability to see.

Of course, Jesus already knew this 2000 years ago, before He ever approached the blind man. He knew the man needed healing of his eyes and his mind.

Why did Jesus choose to heal this man the way he did? Spit,

mud, twice? I have no idea.

I say, Let God be God.

Reading Someone Else's Mail

At some point in human history, God chose to split us up. Out of all the people on the earth, He took one group and separated them from the rest and called them His chosen people. I have no idea why He would do that. As you read the bible, you get the impression that a lot of the time His chosen people may have wanted Him to choose someone else. Hunger, thirst, famine, plague, slavery, wandering around for 40 years. There were also blessings. Provision, victory over incredible odds, great leaders, the advantages of having the Law. The history of His chosen people is full of drama, tragedy, triumph, comedy, irony and all the other elements that make up an epic story. That story was so valuable that God

had some of the
chosen group write it
down. The words God
had them write
became The Old
Testament. A history
and a guide for His
chosen people.
Of course, when you
have a chosen group,
you have an
unchosen group. I am
one of that group.
The term that's used

to describe that group is Gentile, (I think it means "not a Jew", or "without God."

Both the chosen and unchosen groups have the same two parents. Adam and Eve. When they failed, it caused a separation. A separation between mankind and God.

I don't know why God chose to separate Adam and Eve's kids. I do know that the Man that would remove the separation between God and man was born in the chosen group. This Man would reunite mankind and eliminate the two groups. There would no longer be rich or poor, slave or free, Jew or Gentile in the eyes of God. He, Jesus, would reunite all men and women that believe Him.

Now about reading someone else's mail. I consider the Old Testament to be letters from God to

His chosen people. I also think the first 4 books of the New Testament, Matthew, Mark, Luke, and John, are also letters to the same group. Acts through Revelations are a mixture of letters written to both groups, some to the Christian Jews, some to the Christian Gentiles and

Revelations is a letter, written by John, about the future. I believe the entire Bible is valuable and profitable for everyone.

 For some time now, when I read the Bible, I find myself asking, " Who was God talking too?"

We read other people's letters all the time. Family letters written to other family members. Emails we are Cc; on that have, something to do with us, but were not written to us. Letters written by people that are published, interesting because of their historical significance, again not written to us. (Hopefully, we won't be like the postman in the Norman Rockwell painting, taking a peek at other people's mail.) As with all letters, the Bible's letters were written to an intended reader or readers. We, the unchosen, can and

are even encouraged
to read the letters
written to the
chosen. But many
times, the unchosen
choose to think the
letters were written
to them and try to
follow rules and claim
blessings and curses
that were not meant
for them. They claim
a religious history
that is not theirs.

They shape and live their lives based on letters not meant for them. I'm not sure what the dangers are in doing this. I do think there is a loss of freedom that God's Son's sacrifice meant us to have. I do think Gentiles are immeasurably enriched by reading and knowing all of the Bible. It's everyone's history that has ever and will ever be born. It also tells the story of God's love for all of us and the extent He will go to get all of us back.

So, as I read, I always think about what the words I am reading are saying and who

they are saying it to.
If they say, "God
loved the world so
much, that he gave us
His Son. Everyone
that believes what His
Son says and does
will never die and live
forever.," those
words are meant for
me because I am
everyone. If the
words say, "Don't mix
different kinds of

cloth in one shirt," those words were not meant for me. I know this because of where in the bible they are and in what context. The bible is God's words written for all mankind. Some parts are to and about me, much of it is not. It is my job to find the ones that were written to me and do

what it says. The rest
I don't have to worry
about. In that
approach to the bible,
I have found
simplicity, freedom
and salvation.

So go ahead and read
someone else's mail.
Just don't kill your
neighbor if he plants
two different kinds of

vegetables in the
same field.

The Son That Got Lost

Many years ago,
there lived a man that
had two sons. One
day his youngest son
came to him and said,
"Dad, I'd like to get
my inheritance now."
So, his father divided
his wealth and gave
the younger son his
part.

A few days later, the son decided to leave home to find his fortune, so he packed up all of his belongings and started on a journey to a distant country. When he arrived, he immediately began to squander what he had on careless living. In no time, he had spent all he had and began to starve.

There was a famine in the land. Desperately, he searched for a way to feed himself. Eventually, he convinced a pig farmer to hire him to feed his pigs. He was so hungry that even the slop he was feeding to the pigs began to look good to

him, but he was not
even allowed to eat
that.
Finally, he came to his
senses. He thought to
himself, how many of
my father's hired men
have enough to eat.
Here I am, about to
die of hunger. I will
go home. When I get
there, I will say to my
father, "I have
wronged you. I no

longer deserve to be your son. Just make me one of your hired men." So, he got up and went home. When his son was still a good distance away, his father spotted him and his heart jumped in his chest and he immediately took off running to meet his son and when he reached him, he threw his arms around him and kissed him. His son told him what he had planned to say. But before he could finish, his father turned to someone nearby and ordered, "Run and get my best robe and put it on him. Get my ring and put it on his finger and bring him shoes.

Prepare a feast and let's have a celebration. Because my boy was dead, but he came home alive. He got lost, but has been found."
So a great party began.

Now the father's older son was out working in the fields. At the end of the day, as he approached the house, he heard the sounds of a party. He shouted out to someone that was standing nearby and asked him," What's all that noise?" He told him," Your brother has come home, and your father is throwing him a party because he's back home safe."

Hearing this made the older son very angry and he refused to join the party. When his father heard that his son was refusing to come in, he went out too him and asked him to come to the party. But his son refused, telling him," All these years I have done everything you have asked me to do, and not once have I refused. Yet, you have never roasted a lamb for me and my friends. But when this so-called son of yours comes back after wasting everything you gave him on worthless living, you throw him a party." His father responded," My dear son, you have always been at my side and everything I have is yours. But the right thing for us to do is to celebrate your brothers return. He was dead, but he's back home alive. He got lost, but has been found. "

Marriage in Heaven?

I have been thinking about marriage and heaven. The bible says in heaven, we will not marry or be given in marriage. When we love someone here on earth, it is special. It is

separate from all
other relationships.
All our relationships
are different,
whether they are
loving, hating or
somewhere in
between. And it is
true that all loving
relationships differ
from the other loving
relationships we
have. We love our
spouse differently

than we love our kids. We love our parents differently than our friends. It seems to be the way God created us humans. Now I don't know if that was His original plan for us. To have us compartmentalize and differ in degrees the feelings we have for the people we meet as we live our lives.

Adam was created perfect. So was Eve. It makes sense to me that they had maybe the only perfect relationship there has ever been between two people. It couldn't be measured in degrees because it was just them. They had no one else to love so there was nothing to compare their love to. Of course, God was there, but I have no point of reference for how they would love Him. God, being defined as love, could only have loved the two of them with ultimate and perfect love.

But then something came along that would test the happy couples love for God. A nonhuman creature caused Eve to question God's love and good intentions for her husband and herself. The result was that the love relationship between the humans and God changed. We know the love God had for the people He had just created did not change. The love the couple had for God did. The love the two-people had for each other also changed. They were evicted from paradise and were forced to scratch out a life in the wilderness. They

also started to make
more people.

It makes me wonder,
what would their
relationship have
been if they had said
no to the creature.
Would their love for
each other have
remained perfect?
Once they began to
make children, would
their love and their

children's love have remained perfect? As the centuries went by, would the earth have remained a paradise and everyone would love each other? Because perfect love would be what everyone on earth lived, could there ever be a war, or hunger, or sickness or even quarrels

between people?
With universal
perfect love,
everyone would love
God with all their
hearts and minds and
souls. And they would
love everyone and
consider others more
than themselves.
It is hard to imagine
that kind of love
having degrees. With
perfect love, would it

be possible to love your wife more than your neighbor?
I can't imagine people not pursuing special relationships with individual people. I can't imagine not pursuing a woman for the purpose of living life with her and feeling a special love for her. I can't imagine not loving my

children more than
other children.
As we live life on this
testing ground we call
the fallen world, we
enter into special
relationships. We
meet someone we
like and we fall in love
and get married and
promise to live with
that person until we
die, (sometimes we
mean it). Because of

that marriage, children enter our lives and we have a special love for them. We meet people during our life and we form a bond with them and call them friends. Of course, there are the billions of people we will never meet that we have no relationship with except for the fact that we share this earth. We have no feelings for them. Now back to the original thought of this writing. Marriage and heaven.

When Jesus said there will not be marriage in heaven, I wonder if He was saying that there will be no relationships. That's hard for me to imagine. God is a relationship, Father, Son, and Holy Spirit. That cannot be what He was saying. Many people think that we won't even know each other in heaven. We will just be a bunch of people that love each other perfectly. They think we will have forgotten who we were married to and who our family and friends were and who we had special relationships with. Those relationships and special feelings are not possible in heaven due to the fact that we will have the same perfect love for everyone. They say this must be true because there will also be those in heaven we didn't like or that wronged us and hurt us. There can be no memories of those bad relationships either because it would go against perfect love. For heaven to be perfect, I can't love the wife that I lived with and shared everything with for

50 years of marriage and love my neighbor, that I met and became friends with 30 days before I died, with a different level of love.
This is what I think. I believe Jesus was saying that there will not be marriage in heaven because the need for it will end. We won't need to

promise to love someone because it won't be necessary to make that promise. We will just love them. No more need for being married to have kids. (He also said we will be like the angels, which some people have interpreted as "no more sex"). Don't be so hasty! I think the jury is still out on that one. If there is procreation in heaven, marriage won't be necessary because we will always be faithful to each other.

So, the bottom line is, I believe we will carry our relationships with us to heaven. The pain and tears will be removed and we will

see those we loved
on earth with perfect
eyes and perfect
hearts. And we will
love everyone else,
whether we knew
them or not, with
perfect love.

The Stuff We're Made Of

We have known for a long time that everything we can see is made out of the same stuff. Dirt, rocks, trees, animals, bugs, the earth, the planets, the stars, the universe and man. Mankind is made out of the same material as the galaxies. Protons, neutrons, atoms that are just arranged differently depending on what they make up and how they interact. What that means to me is that God had a formula for creation and he used the same ingredients to make everything. Along with making everything out of the same stuff, He determined how it would act and react by creating laws that made everything the way it is and works. The law of gravity, the law of physics. He set the speed limit for light. But there is more than everything, I mean more than the stuff we are made of and the laws that dictate how that stuff works. More than our five senses can detect. We are only limited to how far we can experience this universe by the limitations placed on our bodies and minds

by the laws that
govern them, and by
how far we can
extend those laws.
There is a law that
says, we can't go to
the moon because
there is no air and the
human body needs
air or it will die. But
we discovered that
we can go to the
moon if we take
enough air with us to

last the two-way trip. And we can do it without breaking any laws. What we do is use the material we have to extend our reach into our physical universe. Now think about this. Everything is not everything. Everything that is made of star stuff is not all there is. We know this because we know this. Dirt doesn't know this. Trees don't know this. Animals don't know this. Stars don't know this. The fact that we can think and reason and love shows us we are more than the sum of our parts. There are angels. They are beings that are not made of star stuff. Yet they act and think and communicate. What is really amazing is that they seem to have the ability to move between our physical universe and wherever they call home. From the evidence and what we have learned about them, their main job is to be at

the service of God.
And again, from the
evidence and record,
they're involvement
in human history is
substantial. It has
been said that when
God made man, He
set him apart from
everything else by
giving him a free will.
But I think God gave
the angels the same
free will gift. Before

mankind used his free will against God, an angel used his free will against God. In fact, this angel used the same motivation to tempt our first parents that tempted him. To become like God. And this angel talked a bunch of his fellow angels to go along with his treason. So, God

threw him and his
fellow conspirators
out of heaven, the
place where angels
dwell, and banished
them to earth and the
surrounding area.

Not long after God
placed our first
parents on earth, this
angel successfully
tempted them into
giving up the earth to

him by using their free will against God. And then it got real messy. Brothers started killing each other. A bunch of people started to build a tower to reach God and God had to stop that. Donkeys started talking. People started forcing other people to do their work for them.

It got so bad that God flooded the earth and almost everyone died, except a few people in a boat that had some animals in it. But even after that, man still used his free will against God and those around him. Even though almost everything we did was not what God had intended for us,

God still loved us. He loved us so much that He was willing to pay the price for our restoration to our original perfection and the friendship we enjoyed before we followed that angel's temptation. The price was His Sons life. His Son had to come to earth and be born a man to show us the way back to God and pay the price of our freedom by letting us cruelly kill Him. You can be sure the fallen angel tried to stop Him from doing that anyway he could, but he couldn't stop the Son of God.

So here we are, some 2000 or so years later. Walking talking towers of star stuff, with the option of someday becoming the stuff of angels, if we only believe and live a life that shows it.

By the way, dirt can't believe, trees can't believe, stars can't believe......

What We Do Here On
Earth,
Echoes Forever

The End

www.ingramcontent.com/pod-product-compliance
Lightning Source LLC
Chambersburg PA
CBHW070041210526
45170CB00012B/555